Gabriela Lopes

Pressed ceramics

Gabriela Lopes

Pressed ceramics

Indications and limitations

ScienciaScripts

Imprint
Any brand names and product names mentioned in this book are subject to trademark, brand or patent protection and are trademarks or registered trademarks of their respective holders. The use of brand names, product names, common names, trade names, product descriptions etc. even without a particular marking in this work is in no way to be construed to mean that such names may be regarded as unrestricted in respect of trademark and brand protection legislation and could thus be used by anyone.

Cover image: www.ingimage.com

This book is a translation from the original published under ISBN 978-3-330-20418-8.

Publisher:
Sciencia Scripts
is a trademark of
Dodo Books Indian Ocean Ltd. and OmniScriptum S.R.L publishing group

120 High Road, East Finchley, London, N2 9ED, United Kingdom
Str. Armeneasca 28/1, office 1, Chisinau MD-2012, Republic of Moldova, Europe
Printed at: see last page
ISBN: 978-620-8-33182-5

INDICE

SUMMARY

Aesthetics and function are important factors in restoring dental protection. Various restorative materials have been used throughout history and have undergone structural and optical modifications in order to give the patient something as close as possible to the lost tooth structure. Among these materials are dental ceramics. This literature review aimed to point out the pressed ceramic systems available on the market, as well as the indications and limitations of each one according to each clinical case in the day-to-day dental practice. It was possible to conclude that the clinical longevity of the restorations observed, made with the IPS Empress®, IPS Empress II® and IPS Emax Press® systems, was satisfactory in the literature studied. With regard to marginal adaptation, the maladaptation values presented by the crowns of the IPS Empress®, IPS Empress II® and IPS Emax Press® pressed ceramic systems were lower than the acceptance standard, thus conferring clinical acceptability to these restorations.

Keywords: Pressed ceramics. Ceramic restorations. Ceramic systems. Empress I. Empress II. Emax.

1. INTRODUCTION

Aesthetics and function are important factors in restoring dental protection. Various restorative materials have been used throughout history and have undergone structural and optical modifications in order to give the patient something as close as possible to the lost tooth structure. Among these materials are dental ceramics.

The success of a restoration is linked to its strength, color stability, adequate marginal adaptation, as well as its aesthetic appeal. Ceramics are an alternative for providing the aesthetic, biological, mechanical and functional characteristics required of a restorative material, as well as color stability, biocompatibility and resistance to staining and wear (CARVALHO et al., 2012).

First, ceramic restorations were fitted with a metal infrastructure (metal ceramics), and then *metal-free* ceramic systems emerged with the aim of improving the aesthetics of the work. *Metal-free* restorations can be made with a single layer (monolithic crowns), like glass-ceramic restorations, which are then painted for characterization, or with more layers, where a ceramic infrastructure is made first, followed by the covering ceramic (MARTINS et al., 2010).

In 1930, Carder brought the lost wax technique to the production of glass objects, which led to the development of glass-ceramic systems. In 1958, Vines developed a method for vacuum manufacturing ceramics, making significant progress in this area. As a result, the problem of incorporating air bubbles was considerably reduced (ALVAREZ-FERNANDES et al., 2003).

The quest to increase the strength of metal-free ceramic systems has enabled these materials to be used in the molar region, where the greatest occlusal load is concentrated. In order to increase the toughness of ceramic restorations, a number of changes have been made to their design.

processing, incorporating more elements from the crystalline phase. As a result, various systems have emerged with different reinforcements: silica-based (porcelains and vitroceramics based on leucite and lithium disilicate) and oxide-based (alumina, spinel and zirconium stabilized by itria).

Silica-based ceramics can be reinforced with leucite or lithium disilicate and are represented by the IPS Empress I® and IPS Empress II® systems, respectively (MARTINS et al., 2010). Another pressed system developed was IPS Emax®, with 70% lithium disilicate reinforcement, which has very satisfactory optical characteristics and flexural strength.

In addition to the processing method and structural aspects of each ceramic system, the evaluation of characteristics such as marginal adaptation, mechanical resistance and optical quality become fundamental in determining the indication and limitations of each ceramic material currently available on the market.

2. PROPOSAL

The aim of this study was to review the literature and identify the ceramic systems available on the dental market, their indications and limitations, and their clinical viability and durability as a restorative material.

3. LITERATURE REVIEW

Fradeani et al. (1997) carried out a clinical study in which old/filtered amalgam restorations or teeth with caries lesions in patients with aesthetic needs were replaced with ceramic inlay restorations made with the Empress® system, with the aim of evaluating the reliability of this material in making inlay and onlay restorations in the posterior region of the oral cavity. The study included 29 patients who received a total of 125 ceramic inlays in premolars and molars, the majority of which were molars. Standard-sized cavity preparations were made and the pieces were cemented with dual cement (73% of the pieces) and Variolink® (27% of the pieces), and no significant difference was observed between the results for both cementing agents. The restorations were made using the lost wax technique with stratification and the patients were examined every 6 months for the first year and then once a year for a period ranging from 7 to 56 months. The restorations were evaluated during insertion and at subsequent revisions, where marginal integrity, contour, marginal discoloration, recurrent caries and color change were observed. These characteristics are part of a criterion called "U. S. Public Health Service modified" (Appendix A - Table 1). During the observations, 4 restorations showed fracture-type failure. The longevity of the restorations was almost 5 years in 95% of them, marginal discoloration was within acceptable standards in 65%, marginal adaptation, contour, staining and recurrent caries were satisfactory during the studies. This demonstrated that pressed ceramic inlays and onlays are a viable restorative treatment option.

Sulaiman et al. (1997) compared, in an *in vitro* study, the marginal adaptation of three ceramic systems: In-Ceram®, Procera® and IPS Empress®. Thirty maxillary central incisor crowns (10 for each system) were made according to the processing method of each ceramic system and their marginal integrity was measured during the various stages of fabrication using a digital microscope (Nikon SMZ-U, Nikon). The marginal discrepancy values obtained were 161 ± 46 *um* for In-Ceram®, 83 ± 41 *um* for Procera® and 63 ± 37 *um* for IPS Empress®. As a result, the Procera® and IPS Empress® systems met the acceptable marginal discrepancy criterion of 120 *um.* The lingual and vestibular surfaces showed the greatest degree of marginal maladaptation, while no significantly different values were found between the mesial and distal surfaces. Among the ceramic systems studied, no differences were found in marginal discrepancy during the different manufacturing stages.

Holand et al. (2000), through *in vivo* and *in vitro* clinical studies, compared the microstructure and main properties of the IPS Empress® and IPS Empress II® systems. Ingots of the respective systems (Empress® and Empress II®) were used in the form of restorative infrastructure. After being subjected to pressure and heat (1180°C for Empress® and 920°C for Empress II®), the ingots were injected under pressure into a mold to obtain the ceramic restorations (inlay, onlay, crown or fixed bridge). The microstructure of the restorations was then evaluated using electron microscopy. It was found that leucite is the main component of the crystalline phase of the Empress® system, while lithium disilicate is the main component of the crystalline phase of Empress II®. The flexural strength of Empress II® is 400 +/- 40 Mpa, while that of Empress® is 120 +/-10 Mpa, also showing the high fracture strength of Empress II®. Less wear of the antagonist tooth was observed with Empress II® than with Empress®. The optical characteristics of both systems were satisfactory. *In vivo* tests confirmed the suitability of Empress II® for 3-unit fixed crowns and bridges up to the 2nd premolar. The mechanical properties of Empress II® were superior to Empress®, due to its new microstructure and higher crystalline content compared to Empress®. Empress® can be used successfully in inlays, onlays, crowns and as a veneering ceramic.

Gorman et al. (2000) carried out a study with specimens of two pressed ceramic systems (IPS Empress® and OPC®), with the aim of determining their mechanical properties and differences. In this study, Empress® specimens (Ivoclar®, Schaan, Liechtenstein) were prepared in furnaces at a temperature and pressure of 1180°C and 5 bar, and OPC® specimens (Jeneric Pentron®, Wallingford, USA) at 1150°C and 5 bar. The crystalline phases of both materials were then evaluated before and after ceramic processing by means of X-ray diffraction and electronic images to observe structural changes. Flexural strength was also tested by making disks (2.0 mm in diameter and 1.5 mm thick) using the biaxial method, as well as hardness and fracture resistance using the indentation method. The results revealed that OPC® changes from a mixture of crystalline oxides to a glass ceramic after processing, while Empress® remains a glass ceramic before and after processing. Leucite was the predominant component of the crystalline phase of both materials. The biaxial flexural strength was 153.6 MPa for OPC® and 134.4 MPa for Empress®. Hardness and fracture toughness were 7.28 Gpa and 1.36 (0.29) MPam0.5 for OPC® and Empress®.

OPC®, 6.94 Gpa and 1.33 (0.08) MPam0.5 for Empress®,

respectively. It can therefore be seen that, despite the differences presented by the two systems before processing, the structure of both is quite similar after it is completed.

Brochu & El-Mowafy (2002), through a literature review, analyzed the longevity and clinical performance of ceramic restorations made with the IPS Empress® system. This study was carried out through a Medline survey of articles related to the longevity and performance of IPS Empress® system inlays, onlays and crowns over the last 10 years. The Empress® system material consists of leucite-reinforced glass ceramics, developed primarily for

single-unit restorations (inlays, onlays, crowns and veneering ceramics). The results showed that, in 9 articles evaluated, the longevity of Empress® system inlays and onlays was 96% in 4.5 years and 91% in 7 years. Crowns, on the other hand, had a longevity rate of 92% in 3 years and 99% in 3.5 years. In all cases, the main cause of failure was fracture. It was concluded that the use of IPS Empress® crowns is not indicated in the posterior region until a larger long-term study on premolars and molars is available.

Albakry et al. (2003) conducted a study analyzing specimens from different ceramic systems in order to compare the fracture toughness and hardness of three pressed ceramic systems: IPS Empress®, Empress II® and an experimental ceramic material. For this purpose, 15 disks and 15 bars were made per material, which had their fracture toughness measured using the indentation fracture technique and the indentation forceps, where the hardness of the materials was also measured. The values obtained revealed that there is no significant difference in hardness and fracture toughness between the Empress II® systems and the experimental ceramics, and that the latter have higher fracture toughness and lower hardness than the Empress® system.

Pagani et al. (2003) carried out a study with the
The aim of this study was to analyze the toughness of three ceramic brands: Vitadur Alpha®, In-Ceram Alumina® and IPS

Empress II®. To this end, 10 disc-shaped specimens (5mm in diameter and 3mm high) were made for each system, according to the manufacturing criteria of each. Toughness was measured using the indentation technique, which evaluates the cracks formed when overloaded. A microhardness tester (Digital Microhardness Tester FM, Future-Tech) with a load of 500gf for 10s was used to measure toughness, with subsequent evaluation of the extent of the cracks using a computer program (Image Tool for Windows - version 2.0). The results showed the lowest median toughness value for Empress II® (1.05N/m3/2) and the highest median value for In-Ceram® (2.96N/m3/2), while Vitadur Alpha® showed an intermediate value (2.08N/m3/2). Therefore, the In-Ceram® ceramic system has a greater capacity to absorb stress when compared to Empress II® and Vitadur Alpha®.

In-sung yeo et al. (2003), in an in vitro investigation, evaluated the marginal adaptation of anterior restorations of three metal-free ceramic systems. For this purpose, 120 extracted maxillary incisors (without caries lesions) were prepared for a full crown. Thirty crowns were made for each ceramic system analyzed: In-Ceram®, Celay In-Ceram®, IPS Empress II® and a metal-ceramic control group, in which the respective technique recommended by each manufacturer was used.

Marginal adaptation was measured by measuring the gap between the edge of the crown and the end of the tooth preparation, using an optical microscope and software. These measurements were studied without cementing the grips. The maximum marginal misfit value used as clinically acceptable was 120 *um.* The results showed that IPS Empress II® had significantly less and more homogeneous marginal misfit than the metalloceramic control group. In-Ceram®, on the other hand, showed greater marginal maladaptation and variable dimensions when compared to the control group. There were no significant differences between the Celay In-Ceram® group and the control group. Therefore, crowns made with the IPS Empress II® system showed better marginal adaptation compared to In-Ceram® and Celay In-Ceram®. However, all 3 systems were within the limit value of 120 *um of* clinically acceptable marginal maladaptation.

Ivoclar Vivadent® (2005) reports that, among the metal-free pressed systems, there is IPS Emax Press®, which is a glass ceramic composed of lithium disilicate, obtained using the injection technique. Its microstructure consists of 70% lithium disilicate crystals 3-6 mm long embedded in a glass matrix, giving the system a flexural strength of 400 +/- 40 MPa. The higher strength of Emax Press® and Empress II® compared to Empress® is due to the presence of lithium disilicate in their composition. Another system is IPS Emax ZirPress®, composed of fluorapatite crystals, which contribute to aesthetics by acting on its opalescence. However, its flexural strength is low (110 Mpa), limiting its use to the anterior region and single crowns.

Marquardt et al. (2006) evaluated, through a clinical study, the longevity of ceramic restorations made with the IPS Empress II® system over a 5-year period. The study included a total of 43 patients (19 women and 24 men) who received a total of 58 fixed adhesive ceramic restorations made using the IPS Empress II® system. Of these restorations, 27 were full crowns of molars and premolars and 31 were three-element fixed bridges in the anterior region and premolars. The examinations took place 6, 12, 24, 36, 48 and 60 months after the restorations were placed, and the data was then collected and analyzed. The results showed that the longevity of the crowns was 100% and of the three-element fixed bridges, 70%, with the most common failure in the case of fixed bridges being fracture. However, aesthetically, the results were favorable for both the crowns and the fixed bridges. As a result, it can be seen that the IPS Empress II system is an appropriate material for use in single crowns, while it should be evaluated with caution for use in three-element fixed bridges, given its reduced longevity and the strict conditions in these cases.

Clavijo et al. (2007) presented a clinical case in which a smile rehabilitation treatment was carried out, with the fabrication of 6 anterior-superior ceramic crowns, using the

Emax ZirPress® ceramic system. The 56-year-old female patient's main complaint was the appearance of her smile. There was a metal ceramic crown on tooth 13 and extensive composite resin restorations on teeth 11, 12, 21, 22 and 23.

For this reason, we proposed the fabrication of 6 single crowns using the Emax ZirPress® system (Ivoclar Vivadent®), in order to meet the patient's aesthetic and functional needs. The crowns were made using the injection technique, with a zirconium oxide tablet stabilized by (trio (indicated in cases of teeth with color alteration) and layered with Emax Ceram®. IPS Emax ZirPress® is an aesthetic glass ceramic to be injected into zirconia oxide frameworks, and the IPS Emax Ceram® veneering ceramic (based on nanofluorapatite) is used to layer all the IPS Emax® system frameworks, giving optical characteristics of translucency and fluorescence similar to the tooth structure. This case showed that the Emax® system is a good alternative for restorative treatment, as long as its use protocol is followed carefully, so that restorations last a long time when associated with appropriate adhesive cementation techniques and resin cements.

Stappert et al. (2008) conducted a study using 80 extracted human molars, where preparations were made to receive partial crowns and then indirect restorations were made in different systems. The aim was to investigate the influence of masticatory fatigue on the marginal adaptation of partial crowns made of different ceramic materials. The marginal adaptation obtained between the cast metal prosthesis systems (gold standard), Targis® hybrid composite resin, IPS Emax Press®, IPS Empress® and the Cerec® CAD/CAM system was evaluated. The results showed acceptable marginal fit values between the groups analyzed, although the CAD/CAM system showed a slight compromise in marginal fit.

Wolfart et al. (2009), in their study, evaluated three-element fixed prostheses made with the IPS Emax Press® system (lithium disilicate) for a period of at least 5 years in the oral cavity of 29 patients. Patients in need of anterior crowns (16%) and posterior crowns (84%) took part in the study. A total of 36 fixed prostheses cemented using the conventional or adhesive technique were analyzed. The IPS Emax Press® system uses the lost wax technique, in which a ceramic tablet is plasticized at 920°C and injected into the veneer mold.

Nineteen crowns were cemented with glass ionomer cement (Ketac Cem®, 3M Espe®) and seventeen were cemented with an adhesive system (Variolink II®, Ivoclar, Vivadent®), and no significant difference was observed between the two groups with different cementations. Observations were made after 5, 6, 7 and 8 years, respectively, of the restorations in the mouth. Within the maximum observed period of 8 years, there were 2 complete fractured crowns out of a total of 36 crowns, demonstrating 93% success. Pressed crowns can therefore be indicated as an alternative to metal-ceramic crowns in the posterior region. On the other hand, the fixed prostheses studied require more space for the material, requiring greater tooth wear and weakening the tooth in the long term, when compared to metal-ceramic fixed prostheses. In conclusion, it was observed that anterior and posterior lithium disilicate ceramic crowns have a success rate of 93% after 8 years. These restorations do not pose a greater risk of failure over the period observed, and their behavior is similar to that of metal ceramics.

Medeiros et al. (2009) made samples of the ceramic systems IPS Empress II® (Ivoclar®) and In-Ceram Zirconia® (Vita®), with the aim of evaluating the flexural strength and diametral tensile strength of these materials, for safer indication and use of these systems. Ten bar-shaped specimens (25mm x 5mm x 2mm) were used for the bending test and fifteen disk-shaped specimens (6mm x 3mm) were made for the diametral tensile test. The IPS-Empress II® ceramic specimens were obtained using the lost wax method. The tests were carried out using MTS 810 equipment (Material Test System - USA), with a load of 10kN and a speed of 0.5mm/minute. The results, after statistical tests, revealed a higher flexural strength for In-Ceram Zirconia® (434.17Mpa) compared to Empress II® (230.80Mpa). On the other hand, the diametrical tensile strength of Empress II® (175.41Mpa) was higher than that of In-Ceram Zirconia®

(151.11Mpa). This shows the difference in values between the two properties evaluated, thus demonstrating that the indication of ceramic systems should not be based on an isolated mechanical property.

Jacob et al. (2010) published a literature review on the IPS Empress®, IPS Empress II® and IPS Emax® ceramic systems. The study revealed that the IPS Empress® ceramic system is constantly evolving in terms of its formulation and nomenclature, making it have different compositions and, consequently, different indications. Among the IPS Empress I®, IPS Empress II® and IPS Emax® systems, the latter is more translucent (70% lithium disilicate). IPS Emax® also has superior flexural strength and optical characteristics compared to Empress I® and Empress II®. Respecting the indications, therefore, the IPS Empress® system shows good esthetic results and clinical longevity.

Harder et al. (2010) evaluated the clinical behavior of three-element inlay fixed partial dentures made with the Emax Press® system. Inlay preparations were made according to the principles of the system in 42 patients (21 women aged 20-61 and 21 men aged 24-67), who received a total of 45 restorations. The edentulous space was equal to or smaller than the size of a molar and the inlay fixed prostheses were cemented with resin cement. During the 70-month follow-up period, 60% of the restorations failed and had to be replaced, showing that the clinical result obtained with inlay fixed prostheses made of lithium disilicate ceramic was not acceptable when compared to conventional fixed prostheses and is not recommended in these cases.

Kern et al. (2012), in a study of lithium disilicate ceramic crowns (IPS Emax Press®), analyzed the clinical longevity of 36 IPS Emax Press® crown-retained fixed prostheses in 28 patients with an average age of 47.5 years. Reviews were carried out after 5, 8 and 10 years of use of the crowns with an average observation period of 121 months. Clinical longevity after 5 years was 100% and 87.9% after 10 years. The percentage of success obtained, when evaluating the preserved remnant and the absence of complications, was 91.1% after 5 years and 69.8% after 10 years. The results showed that lithium disilicate crowns had similar longevity and clinical success to conventional metal ceramic crowns. The fractures that occurred during the study were in crowns that replaced molars, suggesting that lithium disilicate crowns are more safely indicated in the anterior or premolar region, which is the manufacturer's recommendation.

Subasi et al. (2012) carried out an *in vitro* study to evaluate the influence of different termination lines and types of ceramic on the marginal adaptation of two ceramic copings (IPS e.max Press®, Ivoclar Vivadent® and Zirkonzahn®, Zirkonzahn GmbH®). Forty models were prepared to simulate receiving mandibular molar crowns, with two different termination lines: chamfer and shoulder. A total of 40 copings (20 for each type of termination) were made and an observer assessed the marginal fit of each one before cementation using a microscope. After the crowns were cemented (with Variolink II® translucent, Ivoclar Vivadent®), a new evaluation was made using a stereomicroscope (Leica MZ16). The results showed that the types of finish and ceramic had no significant influence on the marginal adaptation of the restorations. Both ceramic systems showed marginal adaptation within the clinically acceptable value of *120um.*

Carvalho et al. (2012) wrote a literature review in order to evaluate the indications, marginal adaptation and clinical longevity of different ceramic systems based on lithium disilicate (IPS Emax Press®) and zirconia (Cerec III®, Procera®, Lava® and Everest®). The marginal adaptation values of the ceramic systems discussed were clinically acceptable (24 to *105um*) and their clinical longevity within a maximum period of 10 years was satisfactory.

Farid et al. (2012) investigated in a study the influence of the thickness of the infrastructure and the covering ceramic on the marginal adaptation of IPS Emax Press® crowns (Ivoclar Vivadent®, Schaan, Liechtentein) during the different stages of fabrication. Three stainless steel dies were created simulating a premolar with full crown preparation. The terminations were shoulder-type and 0.8mm (group A) and 1mm (group B) thick infrastructures were fabricated (10 specimens for each group). Marginal adaptation was measured using a 120x stereomicroscope (SZX12 Olympus, Jpan) at four predetermined points and the data analyzed using software (SPSS) and the independent t-test. The marginal *gap* values measured at each processing stage (infrastructure, ceramic veneer and glaze) were 13.5 (+/-1.4) *um,* 33.9 (+/2.3) *um* and 40.5 (+/-1.7) *um* for group A and 14.9 (+/-2.0) *um,* 35.5 (+/-2.2) *um* and 41.3 (+/-2.0) *um* for group B. There was no significant difference in the marginal misadaptation values between the two groups and an increase in misadaptation was observed after the ceramic coating stage in both cases (group A and B). There was no significant increase in maladaptation after the glaze. As a result, it was found that the IPS Emax Press® system crowns have acceptable marginal adaptation and that increasing the thickness of the infrastructure does not promote greater marginal adaptation.

4. DISCUSSION

According to Jacob et al. (2010), the development of ceramics in the dental field has provided significantly satisfactory results in aesthetic therapy and oral rehabilitation. The great importance given by contemporary society to aesthetics, which reflects on their self-esteem, has led several ceramic companies to offer their products. Consequently, given the vast choice of ceramic systems on the market, it is necessary for professionals to be aware of their properties, indications, advantages and limitations, so that they can recommend them safely.

Among the most widely used ceramic systems are pressed ceramics. These consist of solid ceramic blocks that are cast under high temperature and injected under pressure into molds created using the lost wax technique (Pagani et al., 2003). IPS Empress I®, IPS Empress II® and IPS Emax® are pressed ceramic systems available on the market (Jacob et al.,

2010).

According to Holand et al. (2000), the IPS Empress® system meets the aesthetic requirements of inlay, onlay, crown and veneer restorations, with properties such as translucency, color, fluorescence and opalescence that resemble those of a natural tooth. However, its disadvantage is that it is not suitable for fixed bridges due to its inadequate mechanical strength (120 +/-10 Mpa). In agreement, Brochu & El-Mowafy (2002) found that the use of IPS Empress® crowns is not indicated in the posterior region until a larger long-term study on premolars and molars is available. For Fradeani et al. (1997), pressed ceramic inlays and onlays (IPS Empress®) are a viable restorative treatment option.

The Empress II® system, according to Marquardt et al. (2006), is an appropriate material for use in single crowns, but needs to be evaluated with caution for use in three-element fixed bridges. With regard to the flexural and tensile strength of the IPS Empress II® system, Medeiros et al. (2009),

Compared to other systems, the flexural strength of In-Ceram Zirconia® (434.17Mpa) was higher than that of Empress II® (230.80Mpa). On the other hand, the diametrical tensile strength of Empress II® (175.41Mpa) was higher than In-Ceram Zirconia® (151.11Mpa), thus demonstrating that, with the difference in values between the two properties evaluated, the indication of ceramic systems should not be based on an isolated mechanical property. Albakry et al. (2003) state that the IPS Empress II® system has a higher fracture toughness than IPS Empress®. However, Pagani et al. (2003), when comparing the toughness of the IPS Empress II® system to that of In-Ceram®, found that Empress II® had a lower capacity to absorb stress. And in the studies conducted by Gorman et al. (2000), evaluating the flexural strength of IPS Empress®, the values found were similar to those presented by the system's manufacturer, Ivoclar Vivadent® (2005): 134.4 Mpa and 110 Mpa, respectively.

Another pressed ceramic system is IPS Emax Press®, which is made of a glass ceramic composed of 70% lithium disilicate crystals and has a flexural strength of 400 +/40Mpa, superior to IPS Empress® and IPS Empress II® (Ivoclar Vivadent®, 2005). Carvalho et al. (2012) state that ceramics based on Ktium disilicate (IPS Emax Press®) are indicated for making inlays, onlays, overlays, laminated veneers, anterior and posterior full crowns and fixed partial prostheses of up to 3 elements in the anterior and premolar regions. Harder et al. (2010) obtained unsatisfactory clinical results, pointing out that inlay fixed prostheses made of Ktium disilicate ceramic are not viable when compared to conventional fixed prostheses. In contrast, Kern et al. (2012) obtained good clinical longevity results for crown-retained fixed bridges made with Emax Press®. In this study, Ktium disilicate crowns had similar longevity and clinical success to conventional metal ceramic crowns, but the fractures that occurred during the research were in crowns that replaced molars, revealing that Ktium disilicate crowns are more safely indicated in the anterior or premolar region, which is the manufacturer's recommendation. According to Wolfart et al. (2009), Emax Press® three-element fixed bridges can be indicated as an alternative to metal ceramic crowns in the posterior region.

However, the fixed prostheses studied require more space for the material, requiring greater tooth wear and weakening the tooth in the long term when compared to metal ceramic fixed prostheses. In a clinical case involving single crowns made with the Emax ZirPress® system, Clavijo et al. (2007) state that the Emax® system is a good alternative in restorative treatment, as it restores tooth form and function, giving the restorations color, translucency and opacity,

similarly to the tooth structure.

One of the most important criteria used in the clinical evaluation of fixed restorations is marginal adaptation, because the occurrence of marginal discrepancy in restorations exposes the cementing agent to the oral environment, causing it to dissolve, as well as allowing the infiltration of microorganisms (Sulaiman et al., 1997).

In the studies by In-sung yeo et al. (2003), IPS Empress II® showed significantly less and more homogeneous marginal adaptation than the metalloceramic control group. The IPS Empress II® system also showed better marginal adaptation when compared to the In-Ceram® and Celay In- systems.

Ceram®. Subasi et al. (2012), in their *in vitro* study analyzing the influence of different termination lines and ceramic types on the marginal adaptation of two ceramic copings (IPS e.max Press®, Ivoclar Vivadent® and Zirkonzahn®, Zirkonzahn GmbH®),

found that the types of finish and ceramic had no significant influence on the marginal adaptation of the restorations.

In turn, studying the relationship between the thickness of the infrastructure and the covering ceramic in the marginal adaptation of crowns (IPS Emax Press®), Farid et al. (2012) stated that there was an increase in maladaptation after the covering ceramic application stage and that increasing the thickness of the infrastructure did not promote greater marginal adaptation. Carvalho et al. (2012) reported that restorations made with the IPS Emax Press® system had a clinical longevity of 96% at 4.5 years and 91% at 7 years, and that the main cause of failure was fracture. Wolfart et al. (2009) reported a clinical longevity of 93% after an 8-year follow-up of IPS Emax Press® fixed bridges. Several authors have found marginal misfit values for IPS Empress®, IPS Empress II® and IPS Emax Press® pressed ceramic crowns lower than the acceptance standard of up to 120 *um,* thus conferring clinical acceptability to these restorations (Sulaiman et al., 1997; In-sung yeo et al., 2003; Stappert et al., 2008; Subasi et al., 2012; Carvalho et al., 2012; Farid et al., 2012).

The indication criteria for each pressed ceramic system depend not only on the ceramic material, but on a set of factors that will guide the professional in the proper planning and execution of the treatment. It is therefore necessary to know the clinical case, the restorative material, the impression material, a specialized laboratory, and to carry out occlusal adjustment with periodic controls, so that ceramic restorations have longevity and success (Jacob et al., 2010).

5. CONCLUSION

Pressed ceramics are part of everyday dentistry today and, given the vast choice of ceramic systems on the market, it is necessary for professionals to be aware of their properties, indications, advantages and limitations, in order to be able to recommend them safely.

The IPS Empress® system fulfills the aesthetic requirements of inlay, onlay, crown and veneer restorations, but it is contraindicated in fixed bridges and in the posterior region because of its inadequate mechanical strength.

The IPS Empress II® system has greater fracture toughness than IPS Empress® and is an appropriate material for use in single crowns, but should be evaluated with caution for use in three-element fixed bridges.

IPS Emax® has superior flexural strength to IPS Empress® and IPS Empress II® and is indicated for the fabrication of inlays, onlays, overlays, laminated veneers, anterior and posterior full crowns and fixed partial dentures of up to 3 elements in the anterior and premolar regions. The crowns of this system are more safely indicated in the anterior or premolar region, which is the manufacturer's recommendation, and are a good alternative for restorative treatment, as long as their use protocol is followed carefully.

The clinical longevity of the restorations made with the IPS Empress®, IPS Empress II® and IPS Emax Press® systems was satisfactory according to the literature studied. With regard to marginal adaptation, the maladaptation values presented by the crowns of the IPS Empress®, IPS Empress II® and IPS Emax Press® pressed ceramic systems were lower than the acceptance standard, thus conferring clinical acceptability to these restorations.

REFERENCES

Albakry M, Guazzato M, Swain MV. Fracture toughness and hardness evaluation of three pressable all-ceramic dental materials. Journal of Dentistry. 2003 Mar [cited 2015 Jul 16];31(3): 181-188. Available from: http://www.sciencedirect.com/science/article/pii/S0300571203000253

Brochu J-F, El-Mowafy O. Longevity and clinical performance of IPS- Empress ceramic restorations - a literature review. Journal-Canadian Dental Association. 2002 Apr [cited 2015 Jul 16];68(4): 233-238. Available from: https://cda-adc.ca/jadc/vol-68/issue-4/233.pdf

Carvalho RLA, Faria JCB, Carvalho RF, Cruz FLG, Goyata FR. Indications, marginal adaptation and clinical longevity of metal-free ceramic systems: a literature review. International Journal of Dentistry (Recife). 2012 Jan-Mar [2015 Jul 16];11(1):55-65. Available at: https://www.ufpe.br/ijd/index.php/exemplo/article/viewFile/339/318

Clavijo VGR, Souza NC, Andrade MF. IPS e.Max: harmonizing the smile. Dental Press Estetica. 2007 Jan-Mar [cited 2015 Jul 16];4(1):33-49. Available at: http://www.dentalpress.com.br/cms/wp-content/uploads/2008/03/v4n1.pdf

Farid F, Hajimiragha H, Jelodar R, Mostafavi AS, Nokhbatolfoghahaie H. In vitro evaluation of the effect of core thickness and fabrication stages on the marginal accuracy of an all-ceramic system. Journal of Dentistry(Tehran). 2012 June-Sep [cited 2015 July 16]; 9(3):188-94.Availablefrom: http://www.ncbi.nlm.nih.gov/pmc/articles/PMC3484822/

Fradeani M, Aquilano, A, Bassein L. Longitudinal study of pressed glassceramic inlays for four and half years. The Journal of Prosthetic Dentistry. 1997 Oct [2015 July 16];78(4):346-53. Available from: http://www.sciencedirect.com/science/article/pii/S0022391397700416

Gorman CM, McDevitt WE, Hill RG.Comparison of two heat-pressed allceramic dental materials. Dental Materials. 2000 Nov [cited 2015 July 16]; 16(6):389-95. Available from:

http://www.demajournal.com/article/S0109-5641(00)00031-2/abstract

Harder S, Wolfart S, Eschbach S, Kern M. Eight-year outcome of posterior inlay-retained all-ceramic fixed dental prostheses. Journal of Dentistry. 2010 Nov [cited 2015 July 16]; 38(11):875-881. Available from:
https://www.clinicalkey.com/#!/content/journal/1-s2.0-S0300571210001946

Holand W, Schweiger M, Frank M, Rheinberger V. A Comparison of the Microstructure and Properties of the IPS EmpressT2 and the IPS EmpressT Glass-Ceramics. Journal of Biomedical Materials Research. 2000 July [cited 2015 July 16]; 53(4):297-303. Available from:
http://onlinelibrary.wiley.com/doi/10.1002/1097-4636(2000)53:4%3C297::AID-JBM3%3E3.0.CO;2-G/abstract;jsessionid=5B950048248C705ACED36756B20E2D0B.f02t03

Ivoclar Vivadent AG. IPS e.max® Press: Scientific Documentation [online]. Schaan: Research and Development Scientific Studies, 2005 [cited 2015 July 16]. Available from:
http://www.roedentallab.com/downloads/emaxcaddata.pdf

Jacob FL, Martins Jr. M, Archangelo CM, Progiante OS, Cintra LTA, Correa GO. IPS-EMPRESS I, IPS-EMPRESS II, IPS-E.MAX: Compositions, indications and limitations. UNINGA Review. 2010 Apr [cited 2015 Jul 16]; 3():90-100. Available at: http://www.mastereditora.com.br/periodico/20130708_113130.pdf

Kaytan B, Onal B, Pamir T, Tezel H. Clinical Evaluation of Indirect Resin Composite and Ceramic Onlays Over a 24 Month Period. General Dentistry. 2005 Sep-Oct;35(5):329-334.

Kern M, Sasse M, Wolfart S. Ten-year outcome of three-unit fixed dental prostheses made from monolithic lithium disilicate ceramic. Journal of the American Dental Association. 2012 Mar [2015 July 16];143(3):234-40. Available from: http://jada.ada.org/article/S0002-8177(14)61001-1/abstract

Marquardt P, Strub JR. Survival rates of IPS empress 2 all-ceramic crowns and fixed partial dentures: results of a 5-year prospective clinical study. Quintessence International. 2006 Apr [cited 2015 July 16];37(4):253-9. Available from: http://qi.quintessenz.de/index.php?doc=abstract&abstractID=10976/

Medeiros FR, Chaves CA, Schalch M, Cruz CA. Mechanical evaluation of IPS-Empress 2 and In-Ceram Zirconia ceramics. Brazilian Dental Science. 2009 Jan./Mar. [cited 2015 Jul 16];12(1):70-76. Available at: http://ojs.fosjc.unesp.br/index.php/cob/article/view/255/195

Pagani C, Miranda CB, Bottino MC. Evaluation of the fracture toughness of different ceramic systems. Journal of Applied Oral Science. 2003 [cited 2015 Jul 16];11(1):69-75. Available at: http://www.scielo.br/pdf/jaos/v11n1/v11n1a11.pdf

Stappert CF, Chitmongkolsuk S, Silva NR, Att W, Strub JR. Effect of mouthmotion fatigue and thermal cycling on the marginal accuracy of partial coverage restorations made of various dental materials. Dental Materials. 2008 Sep [cited2015 July 16];24(9):1248-57. Available from: http://www.demajournal.com/article/S0109-5641(08)00040-7/abstract

Subasi G, Ozturk N, Inan O, Bozogullari N. Evaluation of marginal fit of two all-ceramic copings with two finish lines. European Journal of Dentistry. 2012 Apr [cited 2015 July 16];6(2):163-168. Available from:

http://www.ncbi.nlm.nih.gov/pmc/articles/PMC3327498/pdf/dent06_p0163.pdf

Sulaiman F, Chai J, Jameson LM, Wozniak WT. A comparison of the marginal fit of In-Ceram, IPS Empress, and Procera crowns. The International Journal of Prosthodontics. 1997 Sep-Oct [cited 2015 July 16];10(5):478-84. Available from: http://www.researchgate.net/publication/13736897_A_Comparison_of_the_M arginal_Fit_of_In-Ceram_IPS_Empress_and_Procera_Crowns

Wolfart S, Eschbach S, Scherrer S, Kern M. Clinical outcome of three-unit lithium-disilicate glass-ceramic fixed dental prostheses: up to 8 years results. Dental Materials. 2009 Sep [cited 2015 July 16];25(9):63-71. Available from: http://www.demajournal.com/article/S0109-5641(09)00205-X/abstract

Yeo IS, Yang JH, Lee JB. In vitro marginal fit of three all-ceramic crown systems. The Journal of Prosthetic Dentistry. 2003 Nov [cited 2015 July 16];90(5):459-464. Available from: http://www.researchgate.net/publication/9034404_In_vitro_marginal_fit_of_thr ee_all-ceramic_crown_systems

Annex A - TABLES

TABLE 1 - Modified USPHS Criteria

Category	Classification	Features
Combination Color	(A)	The restoration matches the color and translucency of the adjacent tooth.
	(B)	The restoration does not match the color and translucency of the adjacent tooth, but it does match the hue of the tooth.
	(C)	The restoration does not match the color and translucency of the adjacent tooth and is not the same shade as the tooth.
Marginal bleaching	(A)	There is no visual evidence of marginal discoloration, which differs from the color of therestorative material or the color of the structure of the adjacent tooth.
	(B)	There is evidence of marginal discoloration at the junction between the tooth structure and the restoration, but it does not penetrate towards the pulp.
	(C)	There is evidence of marginal discoloration at the junction between the tooth structure and the restoration, including towards the pulp.
Carie Secondary	(A)	There is no visual evidence of deep, dark staining adjacent to the restoration.
	(B)	There is visual evidence of deep, dark staining adjacent to the restoration (but not directly associated with the superficial cavo margins).

Anatomical shape	(A)	The restoration continues with the anatomical shape of the tooth.
	(B)	The restoration is discontinuous with the anatomical shape of the tooth, but the material is not sufficient to expose the dentin or the base.
	(C)	Sufficient loss of material to expose the dentin or base.
Adaptation Marginal	(A)	The explorer does not hold when passed between the tooth and the restoration.
	(B)	The crack is not visible, but the explorer catches it; cracks in the edges, exposed enamel.
	(C)	Cracks on the edges, exposed enamel.
	(D)	Clear cracks in the margins, exposed dentin or base.
T exture Superficial	(A)	The surface texture is as good as the surrounding enamel.
	(B)	The surface texture is rougher than the surrounding enamel.
	(C)	There are cracks and fractures on the surface of the restoration.

** (A) Alpha; (B) Bravo; (C) Charlie; (D) Delta*

Source: General Dentistry. 2005;35(5):329-334.

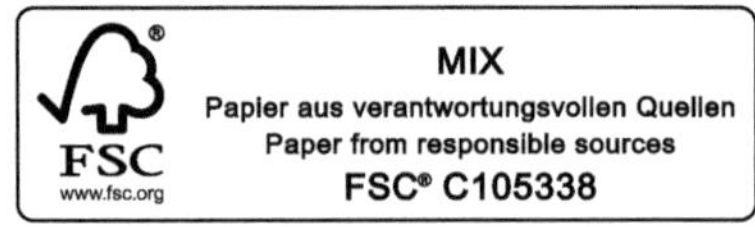

Printed by Books on Demand GmbH, Norderstedt / Germany